The Voices Behind Mental Illness

–

The Mind is a Terrible Thing to Waste

Series 3

Six empowering, encouraging and courageous lived-experiences shared to inspire the world to "Stop the Stigma" around Mental Health and highlight the the "Voices" behind Mental Illness.

FOREWORD BY:

Venessa D. Abram, MBA CPS

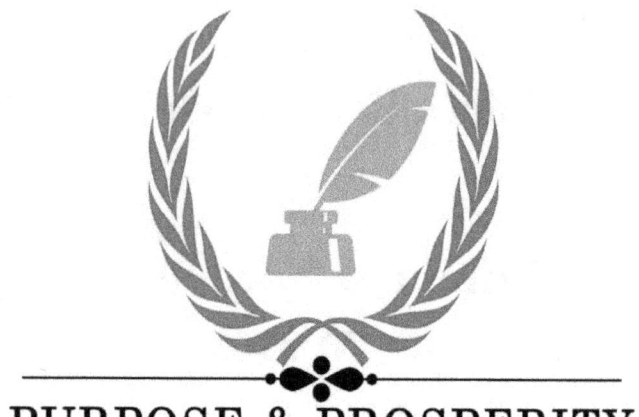

PURPOSE & PROSPERITY
PUBLISHING COMPANY ™

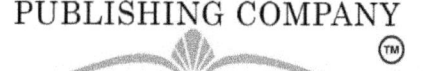

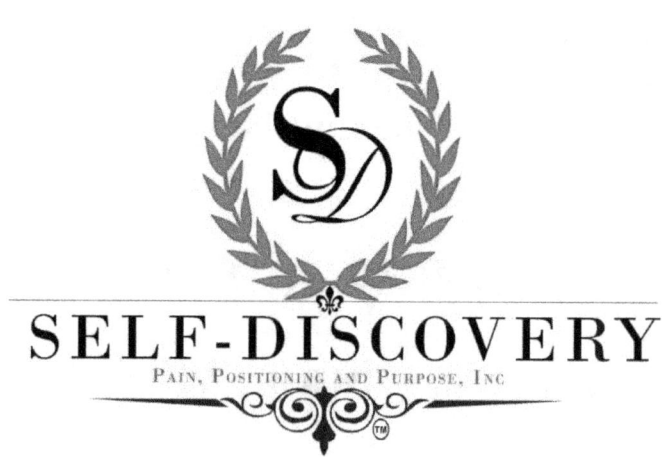

SELF-DISCOVERY
PAIN, POSITIONING AND PURPOSE, INC ™

NATIONAL

SUICIDE
PREVENTION
LIFELINE™

1-800-273-TALK (8255)

suicidepreventionlifeline.org

Dedication Page

This book is dedicated to the Veterans, Soldiers and those perished by way of suicide. Our life and legacy will live on through those of us that boldly and courageously fight the stigma that is attached to mental illness.

You matter. All lives matter.

No Silence. No Stigma. No Suicide.

We are, The Voices Behind Mental Illness.

Table of Contents

Foreword

Mental Health and Suicide is a topic that was not discussed openly in my family. I really never really knew what the true meaning of mental health and mental illness meant until, I attempted suicide the final time. I became very isolated and ashamed that I would act out in certain ways that I personally couldn't understand myself. I tried to keep it a secret that I was taking antidepressants, seeing a Therapist, going to Group Therapy and seeing my Psychiatrist. It wasn't until my last massive bout with Major Depressive Disorder, Anxiety and Post-Traumatic Stress Disorder in 2017 after my brother died. Whom was a decorated Veteran that passed by way of suicide. It was this life experience that I didn't realize would change my life forever. You see, suicide left me broken in ways I could not understand nor articulate. However, having the desire to fight to learn about my struggle and not succumb to it, create opportunities to learn, grow, develop and help others that shared my struggles.

My passion includes fighting by praying God will keep me with every step I take through the day. I ask God to order my steps and to give me my daily bread as I start my day.

Although, I have connected with National Alliance on Mental Illness (NAMI) and become a Speaker, Teacher and Peer-Mentor, I still struggle with suicide ideation. Although, I am on the Junior Board of American Foundation for Suicide Prevention and on the United Survivors International Advisory Board, I still get tired and want to quit. But it is the fact, that I know God has a plan and purpose for my pain, and He will use it for my good and His glory!! It is imperative as a Suicide-Survivor and Sibling-Survivor to continue to *silence the stigma* by sharing my personal lived-experience. It is in sharing my story, others identify with my pain, imperfections, struggles and strain that we are not in this fight alone and mental health does in fact matter. It is in sharing my weakness, others become strong - only through the grace of God. It is in my sharing that I begin to heal, as others heal by way of my truth and transparency.

Destigmatizing the myth of suicide and mental illness is my mission and vision as God open doors of opportunities. Whilst on this journey, it is critical to convey to all we meet that
"The Mind is a Terrible Thing to Waste".

Here are a few nuggets of Self-Discovery:
- ❖ Rid yourself of people, places and things that no longer serve you for the greater good.
- ❖ Allow your pain to position you for God's purpose. There *is* purpose in your pain.
- ❖ Pain results in change. Change results in positioning, and positioning opens the door of purpose.
- ❖ Become a member of NAMI. You will grow in leaps and bounds while learning the fundamentals of mental illness.
- ❖ Stand in your truth and don't become confused about how others perceive you. Someone else's perception of you, is not necessarily your reality!
- ❖ Serve in your community and make the world a better place by sharing your time, talents, gifts and lived-experiences. You Matter! We all Matter.

Venessa D. Abram, Suicide Survivor & Sibling-Survivor

Chapter I.

Anthony L. Abram, Jr.

"Journey to Living Always"

'We don't move on from grief. We move forward with it' – Nora McInerny

October 23rd, 2015 is the day I will forever remember vividly. A day that I wished I could have controlled the outcome. What seemed to be one of the best moments of my life, instantly turned into one of the worst moments of my life. Due to health complications, I never would've imagined this outcome. Everything happened so fast. The day before, after a regular checkup doctor visit. The doctor took her blood pressure, noticing it to be at a stroke level. Which required for us to rush over to the emergency room. After many tests being completed, we were advised that the fluid around the baby was very low. With the fluids around LaMarr being so low, there was a possibility of physical deformity or with mental development delays. My son's mother was suffering from "HELLP Syndrome." Which is very rare. Fewer than 20,000 cases per year. She had been having abdomen pain two days prior, which is one of the symptoms. We thought it was just pain from LaMarr growing, you know not thinking it could be something this severe. Ultimately, it became life threatening for her to continue carrying LaMarr. Due to her liver functions being at an abnormal rate. Her blood platelets count was very low.

When the doctors were explaining it to us it sounded as if he was talking in foreign language. I heard every word but couldn't understand how things got so severe. Doctors then gave us three options. First option was for her to carry LaMarr and risk both of their lives. Second option, was pretty much an abortion. They were going to chop the baby and use a vacuum type of machine to get the remainder of him out, which could cause enough damage for her not to be able to have another baby. Third option, was to have a labor induction.

I felt as if I couldn't make this choice because it wasn't my body being affected. However, I knew we had to have this conversation collectively as one. She wanted to continue to carry our son with great reasoning on why. I thought that the labor induction would be a great idea. I was positive about it. I didn't want to lose both of them. So, we agreed on the labor induction. Around 3:30 pm on October 23rd, my son LaMarr Abram was born into the world at 22 weeks. No crying, no movement. My flesh, my boy, laying lifeless after coming out of the womb. I've seen videos on social media along with movies that had babies coming out crying. I didn't understand. The nurses advised that due to the force trauma of him coming out the womb he didn't survive because he was so little. He was under one pound. LaMarr was small enough to fit into a doll clothing. I was numb from all feelings and emotions after shedding some tears with my family.

Even though I didn't carry LaMarr like his mother did, I still felt the connection. I felt and still feel as if I'm missing a part of me. A part of me that I'll never get back physically on this earth. Seeing him afterwards was tough but I needed that closure. Even though he was still developing he looked just like me. I do know he's always watching over me and moving with me each day.

For about a year and a half, I began to lose myself. I knew I didn't feel like myself. I was more fatigued than ever. I was gaining weight. My mood was always up and down. I found myself faking to be okay most of the time. I would have a cup of liquor every day. I was depressed. When family and friends would call to check on me to ask how I was doing, I'd simply say each time "I'm good" or "I'm okay." Truly knowing I wasn't. Looking back, I was killing myself slowly. Killing myself trying to withstand the image of a man that society has placed on us men, especially black men.

Society says with how we were raised; we have to be strong and not to seem weak by showing emotion. Growing up playing sports, you had to fight, be strong, and show toughness. If you fall and scratch your knee during a basketball game, you were told to "Get it up, there is no crying, keep going." We're trained so early to uphold this image. So, when life hits us the hardest, we are still trying to hold on to this image. Well society will have us all killing ourselves by trying to operate that way. I slipped into an all-time low point, by trying to be strong to prove that I was a man. I didn't know any better. No one in my family had ever experienced an infant death before, so who could I relate to? I didn't believe in speaking with a therapist at the time. I felt that God would handle everything for me. Even without me trying to help myself as he worked too. Surely, I had to put in work on myself as well. My son's mother always suggested I speak with a therapist. I always shot the idea down as well. I noticed everything else coming together in my life, still mentality I wasn't right.

It ultimately came down to me being tired of the space that I was in. I had to make some lifestyle changes to get back to feeling and being me. I first started eating healthier and working out more. Then I started reading self-help books to find inspiration and motivation. Lastly, I sought therapy. Seeking therapy was the best thing I could've done. I was able to just talk and express how I felt, while my therapist just listened. She would listen and take her notes, then hit me with a follow up questions that made me think deeper into my feelings. Which made me vulnerable to expressing myself, in a way society told me not to. I tapped into a new level of me I never knew I had before therapy. Since then my communication level has increased especially with truly expressing my feelings. Therapy has been beneficial for me. I'm more than positive it would be beneficial for you, too. Now I can identify when I need to go back to therapy. I seek the help before I cause myself to stress or slip back into the place, I once was in. I hold myself accountable for my overall health. Especially, my mental health which is number one.

It's almost been four years now since LaMarr's passing. Since then I've been trying to find my purpose with sharing my story to the world. In 2017, is when I launched my Blog Site, "Living Always". The title comes as a representation for LaMarr's name. I blog on topics around mental health and pregnancy loss awareness, along with putting positivity into the universe. Also, the main goal of *Living Always* is to keep him living through my purpose of speaking on my situation and inspiring people to leave their own legacy that will be living always. It doesn't matter your age or where you are in life you can still leave a legacy that will be living always. I'm finally in a good overall space to share my story. It's been two years of just putting out Blogs, trying to find the right approach to launching my business as well. It's been a marathon for sure. I thought initially it would happen overnight, I'm glad it didn't because my story wouldn't have been the same. Nevertheless, I've been able to find my purpose through my pain. It's more for you to go through and grow through for you to reach your purpose.

Today, I continue to seek treatment for myself. Other factors in life can cause stress which can lead to depression or anxiety. For me, I tend to get anxiety. Anxiety for me comes from the cognitive distortions - those negative thoughts trigger my anxiety. The past year more specifically with my finances triggered me seeking therapy again. For the first time I wasn't the breadwinner in my relationship. When I didn't have it, my anxiety kicked in. I would shut down. I wouldn't communicate properly. Which caused unnecessary arguments and stress on my significant other. Again, how society labels us as men, I let pride get in the way of communicating. We're always supposed to be able to take care of home, is how society paints us. Sometimes we can't always be superman and save the day. At times we're going to need our wonder woman to come in and help us out. If you are suffering from a pride issues with anything, let it go for the greater good of your spouse. It wasn't right or acceptable, but I had to seek help.

Since seeking the second round of therapy, I've still been working on turning those negative thoughts into positive thoughts. Reminding myself I can control my thoughts even though it's a rough patch, there is a lesson in everything we go through. I must remind myself that I am okay in the current space I'm in. Moreover, life will continue to be a marathon with highs and lows. No matter what you can dictate how you finish the race, by simply asking for help.

I encourage anyone that has went through any loss, depression, anxiety or suffering from any mental illness to use these tips above. Along with tips throughout the book to get proper treatment and help. Your situation doesn't define you. It's just a humble piece of your story. Along with building a stronger, wiser you. Giving up it's not an option! Fight the fight, you'll win the fight! There is light always at the end of the dark tunnel! It's takes courage, so be courageous about your journey! I had to tell myself that my story and journey may impact one person. That's all I need. It's way bigger than me. Sharing this story is difficult, however it's necessary for me. I made it to this point that we must end the stigma. We must work together as one to help one another. If you've been through the dark storm and made it out, you have a voice to provide to someone that's entering the storm. You are the courage and inspiration someone needs. For me, I didn't move on from grief. I moved forward with it.

Map to Mental Wellness Success

Ladies it is never your fault for the loss. Do not try to take the blame for what is out of your control.

Gentlemen never make the mother feel as if it's her fault for the loss. Always reassure that she knows when she is expressing her feelings.

Ladies and Gentlemen talk about your feelings amongst each other. Openly sit down and express how you're really feeling.

Try seeking therapy together. Be open. Maybe doing therapy together will make it more comfortable for each other to talk about.

Invest in yourself. Seek the proper help to elevate yourself to a better you mentally. Which will translate to an overall better you.

Do not hold in bottled up emotions. Talk about how you really feel. Do not hide your emotions.

Do not use drugs and alcohol as a method to cope with your loss.

Speak up and Speak out!

Anthony Abram Jr.

Anthony is a 26-year old Indiana native but currently resides in Atlanta, GA. Anthony is the creator and owner of *Living Always*, along with a speaker on the SD PPP 'Taking off the Mask: International Mental Health Tour 2019'. Living Always was developed in 2017, it is devoted to spreading mental health and pregnancy loss awareness, along with inspiring everyone to leave a legacy that will be living always. Anthony's goal is to use his life experiences as motivation for others, reminding everyone they can overcome their current and/or past situations.

This chapter is inspired and dedicated to his son and his step-mother's grandson in heaven,
LaMarr Abram.

Website: www.livingalways.org

Chapter II.

JoAnne Nichole' Brice

"I've Decided to Talk About IT"

Jeremiah 29:11 "For I know the plans I have for you,' DECLARES the Lord, "plans to prosper you and not to harm you, plans to give you hope and a future" (NIV)

Ever had that moment or feeling you just can't take anything else? Do you fold, lay in the dark being non-productive, or do you open up, let it out, heal and impact the world? **I'M GOING TO IMPACT THE WORLD!!** I didn't think I had anyone to reassure me of who I am, nor what I am worth. That left a lot of room for mistakes, heart aches and let downs. I am the apple of God's eyes and knowing who I am in God and what I am called to do – makes all the difference.

Day one of my life: Mommy was fifteen and she was not allowed to put my Daddy's name on my birth certificate. I was born... a stigma. Daddy wasn't "good enough" and the family of "the other dad" had a good name for themselves. Don't people make you sick sometimes?! Meanwhile, Daddy has held four jobs my entire life; a police officer, a teacher, a Principal and now retired he is a consultant for Delaware State University. He caters on the side and has built a car. He is actively working on two, '55 Chevy and a '68 Camaro. The older I got, the more I started to look like Daddy and not the dad I was forced upon. I started feeling resentment from him and some of his family. Finally, he just stopped coming but Mommy never stopped sneaking me to see Daddy. I loved going to Grandma's house because my great -grandmother had a salon and I would sit in there with her for hours. Some of my best days happened in that house on Tilghman Street in Oxford, Maryland.

When I was seven, Mommy started dating this guy, and it wasn't long before he became very abusive to her. Scared to death, I would go lay in the bed listening to Mommy getting verbally abused and thrown against walls like a little rag doll after she came home from work at 11pm. That never stopped her flow. Every day, she got up early to carry him to work, came back home, and got my sister and I ready for school. She took us, came home got dinner together, and cleaned the house, laid our clothes out, then got her rest for work. She always picked us up from school, checked our bags, dropped us off to Grandma's, and if something wasn't right, we were getting up at 11pm when she got off to fix it.

When I was ten, he beat Mommy breaking seven ribs, her ankle, bit her face, choked her to unconsciousness... leaving her for dead and walked to police station. The officer he was looking for was off that night. He went back to Mommy and found her conscious, he beat her back unconscious for someone else to find her. At any given moment, I can still see the visual of her laying in the hospital bed. Mommy had a restraining order against him and he still beat her the way he did. Mommy loved him.

When I was thirteen, I planned to get up because I needed help with my homework. I couldn't sleep because I was having real bad pains in my body and chest. I woke my

Grandma up because Mommy was getting home late; Grandma told me she was probably out partying. I fell asleep hours later my Aunt Inez woke me up to tell me he had killed my Mommy at her job in the parking lot. EVERYTHING changed!! Everyone in the house separated. Everyone was hurt to the core with no direction on how to handle it. As much as Mommy used to take us to visit the other family, none of them came to check on us. Of course, once we were grown, everyone wanted us to come spend time with them. The years I needed them… they abandon me – child cheese. I'll see 'em when I see 'em. I don't even know you to trust you with my children. GET!

Fourteen years ago, I forgave that man…Herbert. I have never been to any of his hearings because we were never contacted when he had them. In August 2017, he sent me a book with a spine on it directly from the jail telling me how he planned for two days to kill Mommy. He pretty much confirmed he set our house on fire with my sister and I in it and plenty I didn't need to know.

Once I reported it to the Karen Green the Domestic Violence Coordinator for Talbot County, her response was not to except any more mail from him. He is crazy! She took a phone call about a domestic violence incident over the weekend, got off the phone, walked to her secretary and said, "I got all the scoop!" She escorted me out the office. So, once again, the victim is victimized by the very person I thought had things in place so that he couldn't contact our family. I ended up going to the Attorney General's Office who assigned a mediator to me. I sat at the table and explained everything. Sometimes you just have to look the devil in the eye to tame him.

I turned to boys and at age nineteen I had my first son. After telling his father I was pregnant that was it! He turned into Casper the Friendly Ghost. When my Son was nine months old I met Joey. He was thirty-one. We started dating five months later and he got us a place. I thanked God for him, because he was truly a blessing to our son. I finally was at peace. I felt worthy, loved, confident, and I felt SAFE. Joey had a way of building up my confidence. He always made our little family a priority. There wasn't anything I ever wanted for and that old bird taught me a lot. After twelve years we broke up, but we never were on bad terms and he never stopped being a part of our world even after I had other kids. We both eventually married other people, but he never left our son. In November, 2005 Joey was murdered. The love of my life who I had just spoken to the night before, was gone. We just had lunch with him two days prior to his death. That was it... now, the two people who loved me the most were gone.

On January 25th of my 39th birthday, I asked God to reveal myself to me! Why did I do that? May of the same year, my sister texted me a question. I responded. I looked at a plain white wall and God was showing me a movie (revelation). He showed some things I suppressed, due to the trauma of Mommy's death back to my remembrance. Two major things: the woman who molested my sister and I and a man calling me to reveal that he was actually my grandfather. He actually called in 1999 and I shared this with my grandmother. Grandma told me to call the police someone was trying to scam me…lol. I just didn't pay it any mind. However, God showed me in another dream ten years later that confirmed that call. I got a picture of the man that called me and saw my mommy and my aunt's faces in his. All of her siblings knew of her. Everybody around us knew, however, nobody thought it was robbery not to share it with my sister and I. I also was able to understand why I was rejected after mommy passed – I didn't belong. However, my grandfather died by then so I never got a chance to meet him…all because of a lie.

I shut myself off to the world except for one persistent young lady that would not leave my side, Lisa Michelle Hayman (Woolford) to this day, if she is rockin', I'm rollin'! Sometimes I think she knows me better than I know myself. I met her because she is my cousin on the "other daddy's" side. Too funny! She never treated me any different! Her father was the 'other daddy's" brother; he and his wife treated me as if I was their niece. They did not take someone else's poor decision out on me like so many others were doing. The stigma just continued on as I got older for one thing or another. Generational curses are what they are called.

That doesn't even cover half of what I have been through. Due to a lot of the trauma, I have a diagnosis of Bipolar, Depression and Anxiety. Let me define Bipolar for those that really don't know what it is or are reading it out of a book. We love harder than average, which makes our response more intense as well. My psychotherapist doesn't necessarily like to place a diagnosis on people. She is fully aware of what the book definition says, however, in my opinion, her relationship and trust in the Lord is going to help deliver 90% of her patients. She doesn't speak such labels in the air, nor did she really want me to put it in this chapter. The stigma the world tries to place on us who have been through hell and high water and know we are hurting but are determined not to live in this pain. How can your mood not swing with all the experiences you have had in conjunction with what's going on around you today?

For example, the police stopped me the other day and searched my car in front of my salon after I saw the cop touch my car to make the dog alert. I have to be respectful because my son was with me and I have taught him how to act, so I need to act accordingly. Four days later I had a nightmare that the police and I were on a high-speed chase and they were trying to kill my son and I was calling Joey (who always protected me) to come and meet me before I stopped the car. Of course, he never answered as he has been dead for fourteen years. I woke up beside myself. On top of that a bad company so called fixed my refrigerator with a penny with a hole in the center. Due to that, I lost another refrigerator full of food. While all of this was going on, I'm still not working due to a car accident.

It was Mother's Day, and for whatever reason this year, I was sick of people celebrating their Moms. Selfish... I know! That's just how I felt. I have anxiety because I have to get a steroid shot in my back to help me move my arms and gain strength in my elbows. All of this is actively going on while I'm attempting to write this chapter. I have had my melt downs, I have stayed to myself, and I couldn't take a slick selfie if I tried! I decided to get head shots taken.

Shamya Lynne Studios just made my day! She was having a bad day as well, but still did what she needed to do to help me have the best photoshoot ever.

That evening, I was on facetime with my girlfriend Von, she looked at me over her glasses like her Grandmother Catherine (Skittles) used to do and asked me one question. I needed to pray and that's what I did. I woke up in the middle of the night with revelation and was able to dig up a root just by admitting it existed.

I used to wonder why I have been chosen to go through so much dysfunction and why many things leave permanent marks in my mind. I need to have experience to help someone. Someone is going through mental issues and doesn't want to tell anyone. They don't want people to call them names or make them feel less than. Allow them to talk about getting help and not getting you out of jail or a mental institution. Your mental health is just as important as your physical health, if not, more important. Without your mental health being stable, how can you function properly physically or emotionally? People are going to talk if you do good or if you do bad, so you might as well shine. I am no longer going to fight this alone and I suggest you don't either. Be honest and tell people if you don't want to be bothered. Please... if you need to cry – CRY! Crying is a healing mechanism. It also recharges you to take the next steps forward.

Map to Mental Wellness Success

- Find a therapist(s) that works for you. You may go through a few, however, do not get discouraged. This is for you! We fire the nail tech or the suit tailor for less, fire the therapist. Allow your mind to be worth more than that.

- Take time for yourself and whatever gives you peace, do it often.

- Learn to say **NO!** That word helps people make their own way and relieves pressure off of you.

- Your truth is yours. People may not harm you intentionally, but it doesn't change the hurt you feel. You are allowed to express that. If they don't respect it, you are allowed to walk away without being angry. Again, sometimes it just has to be about **YOU** when it comes to Mental Health.

- Confide in someone you trust and be honest about what you go through…we need all the sincere prayers we can get.

- Get your relationship with God in order… Not the rules of religion, but an actual relationship with God and watch how things turn around for you.

- Hiding and shaming yourself adds to the issues we already have – free yourself! Own it and go. Do what you have to do to keep you at a level of peace, joy and comfort.

- Seek support groups to help others, as well as gain tips from other survivors or others that are maintaining.

- I see a therapist (Dr. Whitehead, Reflective Image Counseling, Inc) and a Psychotherapist (Dr. Barrett, Triumph Behavior Health) located in Catonsville, Maryland. They work together so everyone is on the same page. Try them out if you're in the local area. Whatever you do, please make sure everyone is on the same page. You don't need anything else frustrating you and you want to be allowed to fight for you.

Continue surviving… JNichole

JoAnne Nichole' Brice

JoAnne is from Easton, Maryland. She is first a mother to Jahleel, Jahsua, Jahtera, Amber, Erin, Lakia (Reese), Catonya, Glynna, Shyann and twelve grandkids. JoAnne is a Senior Cosmetologist, who is passionate about her craft and focusing on healthy hair. She is an Author and a Voice for Domestic Violence, forgiveness, and Mental Health Awareness. Naturally, she is a motivator and encourager, she often pushing her issues aside to make other's joy come alive. With that infectious smile she has, how can she not? For far too long she has received people speaking ill over her life. JoAnne no longer receives it; SHE IS ON ASSIGNMENT!

She lives life based on *Jeremiah 29:11 "For I know the thoughts that I think toward you, saith the Lord, thoughts of peace, and not of evil, to give you an expected end."* JoAnne is a reflection of love.

Contact JoAnne here: www.Joannenichole.com

Chapter III.

Daphkar Dubreuil

"Monuments of the Mind"

"No difficulty can discourage, no obstacle dismay, no trouble disheartens the man who has acquired the art of being alive. Difficulties are but dares of fate, obstacles but hurdles to try his skill, troubles but bitter tonics to give him strength; and he rises higher and looms greater after each encounter with adversity." - Ella Wheeler Wilcox

We have all been enamored with the idea of instant gratification, regardless of the physical or mental consequences that it has to offer. Mental illness and our everyday complexities are no less different. For so long, I yearned to experience a place where this fear and worry could no longer cripple my daily life. We often take ourselves and our minds for granted, and we don't realize how much we can handle, until handling it is the only option we have. At the simple age of fourteen, I found myself perplexed with the idea of having to take a simple midterm exam in high school, and that anxiety continued to slowly creep up on me through the years. I gradually felt myself shifting with the way I would process certain things.

My confidence was dwindling, and my ability to handle every day circumstances became a greater mountain to climb. After some time, the excessive worry resonated with me so profoundly that I could not even leave my house unless it was for something urgent, and I stopped driving entirely. Throughout my sophomore year in college, I continued to experience horrific physical symptoms which only progressed from my high school days, and left me wondering if this is how I would forever be. I was nauseous all the time, my whole body would get so stiff it would be stuck and extremely painful; I experienced weight loss, hair loss, muscle stiffness, nausea and vomiting constantly. I took advantage of the fact that my sister and I were attending the same university; therefore, she would attend all of my classes with me on top of her sixteen credits courses in order for me to not have a panic attack.

Anxiety can creep up on us in so many ways, and if we are not guarded it can allow our minds to run rampant despite our best efforts. Pretty soon, I found myself having to take a break from school in order to recollect and allow myself the space to get back to a place that I once was. I had to let go of ego, perfection, fear, worry, and always wanting to please those around me. These are the internal battles that many of us face or will face at some point in our lives. During this break, I found myself seeking answers to what I was experiencing. I was not at all where I wanted to be in life, and I was watching all my friends move on, continuing their educations, and accomplishing all the goals that they had set out to accomplish during their college tenure.

This put me in even more of a rut and I couldn't see the light at the end of the tunnel. I had an idea that it was anxiety because every little thing would worry me to the point of an anxiety attack, and it greatly interfered with my daily activities. I could be eating dinner and I would have an anxiety attack out of nowhere, even if i wasn't thinking of anything triggering; at the end of it all, I was anxious all the time and I knew that I wouldn't be sure what it was until I spoke with a professional. Often times, we are so afraid of stigma or being judged that we would much rather carry our mental or physical baggage in order to "look the part" in the eyes of the world around us.

This began to gnaw away at me until I found myself on Google seeking for help, and seeing if there were others like me going through what I was going through. The ideology of reaching rock bottom mentally became so strong in my mind that I had to seek help. I began expressing my worries and fears to someone professionally, and in return, they gave me the necessary tools to channel these fears and these worries into something positive. It also allowed me, for the first time, to realize just how much the internal dialogue we have with ourselves is real. Our minds are a manifestation of excellence. I realized through speaking up that I could either build monuments of self-awareness, honesty, and accountability or I could choose to remain stagnant with where I was.

One of my biggest motivations was the openness of those around me sharing their own personal issues with mental health to me. This included mentors, peers, classmates, family and friends. They began to express to me just how much my willingness to be open with my personal struggles, allowed them the platform to do the same for themselves. This experience granted me the opportunity to recognize that mental health is not black and white, and it most certainly does not discriminate, regardless of who you are. It comes in all different forms, from minor to severe. It took me a total of seven years before I would come to acknowledge the issues that I was struggling with, and I remember vividly when it all began.

I can point to so many occasions where I recognized that it was gradually increasing, but the stigma kept me from speaking up. We would never shame an individual for having something as minor as a cold, to something as extreme as cancer, and we wouldn't shame them either for seeking professional help in order to alleviate their illnesses as best as they can. Therefore, I had to learn to not shame myself for choosing to fill my cup and I had to do whatever was necessary to become the best person that I could be.

Map to Mental Wellness Success

I became my biggest advocate and I regulated any thoughts of validation that I was seeking from anyone other than myself. I am living proof that mental health comes in an array of intensity, and the earlier we seek to condition our mind, be-it individually or professionally, the sooner we can continue aligning ourselves with purpose. If we are not cautious in caring for our mental health while it is well, we create a gateway to allow room for mental illness to occur. Like I've mentioned before, mental health is not black and white, and there are many facets to it; therefore, it behooves us to know that we can still at any given time become prone to developing a mental illness. However, the absence of mental illness does not invalidate caring for our mental health. There is a plethora of positive coping strategies both physically and mentally that will enable us to sustain great mental health. I had to put in the work mentally in order to see the results come to fruition. I challenged myself daily in therapy by starting from the ground up. I expressed my thoughts every day, both good and bad and put pen to paper.

I also indulged in practicing mindfulness which led me to studying what my habits were so that I could identify and deal with negative patterns. I promised myself that I would "stop and smell the roses" because I had to remember that life was and is a gift that should never be taken for granted. I began monitoring my mental exposure so that I would understand what things would enhance triggers that would put me in a compromising position. Don't get me wrong, working towards something we truly value or want is never easy, but there is a beauty in consistency. It allows our mind to experience a form of mental stability while developing our emotional stamina to prepare us for whatever life has to throw at us.

Conquering and conditioning the mind is the one of the hardest things we will ever have to do because it is the center of our personality, our cognition, and it dictates our behavior. The physical and the mental are both connected, and our bodies are machines that combine every part to produce a fully functioning individual. One of the biggest misconceptions that we often face is that self-care and maintaining a positive mental health is easy, but it is far from it. It takes courage, strength and dedication to recognize that some of the things we expose ourselves too, also assist in our greatest anxieties. For me, I've had to examine all that I was doing both physically and mentally that contributed to what I started to experience.

Working on ourselves will be the greatest accomplishment and legacy that we can leave behind, it is about making a difference and being aware of how we make others feel around us. We do not have to wait until there is an issue to take our health seriously, prevention is crucial to maintaining a positive mental health. The mind is a machine that we have to constantly get a "tune up" for in order to know that we are on the right track, so we won't breakdown from lack of care. You are not your mental illness, and you are not whatever circumstances you may face. We are all connected and bonded by the human experience. Never be ashamed to speak up for yourself and for those who can't.

Mental illness is very common, and mental health now more than ever is truly important. We must access and acknowledge the emotions that we feel. Allow yourself to feel whatever it is you need to feel, and do not bow your head in shame for whatever it is that it may be. The mind is a terrible thing to waste, from it comes our ability to think, feel, and act and I truly hope that we continue to appreciate life, and know that each and every one of us are worthy of good things and a good life.

Daphkar Dubreuil

Daphkar is a Mental Health Advocate and the Founder of Anchors 2 Oasis, a Mental Health Organization which seeks to eradicate the stigma surrounding mental illness, specifically in the community of African-Americans. She graduated from Florida Atlantic University, where she received her B.S in Neuroscience and Behavior. She also graduated from Lynn University with her M.S. in the field of Psychology. Her mission is to allow others to recognize and unlock their full potential by educating themselves on mental health, and how it ultimately affects who we are, and the world in which we live in.

Email Daphkar: ddubreui444@gmail.com

Chapter IV.

Monique A. Lynch

"Using FEAR to Fuel Success and Purpose"

Fear and Disobedience are two of the deadliest killers of success and purpose-

Like many people, I am terrified of snakes, especially the Anaconda; they are huge, aggressive and will attack and eat you without provocation. But many of us including myself have never seen an Anaconda before and watching it on television is as close as we will ever get to a live one. So, how do we develop a fear of something without ever seeing or experiencing it?

Fear can be a temporary feeling, but it can also be a permanent one. In many instances, it can control your life, affect your daily functioning such as difficulty sleeping, eating, concentrating, and being productive or progressive (leaving the house or going to work or school). Fear can really prevent you from doing things you want or need to do, and it also affects your health. For some people they can be so fearful that they intentionally avoid circumstances that might make them fearful or anxious. It is very hard to overcome fear, but there are mental wellness tips that I will share on how to achieve this.

Luckily, most fears are learned. Fears can, therefore, be unlearned by practicing self-discipline repeatedly regarding fear until it goes away. The most common fears that we experience, which often prevents and delays all hope for success and purpose, are the fear of failure, poverty, not being perfect before God can use you and loss of finances. These fears cause people to avoid risk of any kind and to reject opportunity when it is presented to them. They are so afraid of failure that they are almost paralyzed when it comes to taking any chances at all.

There are many other fears that interfere with our happiness, success or fulfilling our purpose.

- People fear the loss of love or a relationship
- People fear the loss of their jobs, businesses and their financial security.
- People fear being embarrassed or ridiculed.
- People fear being rejected and criticized in any way.
- People fear losing the respect of others.
- People fear being challenged or placed outside their comfort zone
- People fear pursuing purpose at the expense of their own desires

These and many other fears hold us back throughout life and prevent us from being successful and purposeful.

My Testimony

Growing up, throughout primary school (grades 1-6), I have always been a brave and smart child. I always came in the top three every school year, I was popular among the students, I was favored by the teachers, and life was great until I gave my life to God in April of 2005 and that's when everything changed for the worse. I started having trouble dealing with fear as I didn't know who I was in Christ, I didn't know my purpose and without purpose, I was a guideless fool. I had a strong calling on my life, I knew I was a leader, but the fear of leading turned me into a follower. There wasn't a minor that I couldn't turn into a major. I missed out on many opportunities that would have really changed my life because of fear. I would sit at the back of any session, I would have a minor panic attack if I was to present in front of any audience, even to introduce myself and when I do, the words would disappear and it was like fear had paralyzed me.

When I transitioned into early adulthood, fear turned into worry and doubt. I was always worried about bills, money, this problem, that problem until even the word of God that I knew was the ultimate truth, I doubted it. I realized that it is easier to be fearless when you are in your comfort zone, but when my life demanded faith, I chose fear. Everything we do is either wrapped around faith or fear. So how do use fear to fuel our success and purpose?

I am who I am today because I have mastered fear and used it to pursue my calling and purpose in life through the strengthening of my faith, knowing who I am, finding my purpose and being the best version of myself. I was twenty-three-years old, divorced, depressed and lost so I crawled back to the throne of God and recommitted my life. This time, I took the opportunity to know God in a different way, I prayed, fasted and read the word of God more so I grew and as I grew, my faith was strengthened. Additionally, my faith was maintained through having like-minded people around me to mentor, advise and encourage me.

Knowing who you are is the greatest wisdom any human can possess. So, I took the time to introspect, self-reflect and got to know myself, the real me. I had to figure out what my goals were, what I loved, my morals, my needs, my Godly standards, and what I will not tolerate, what I was willing to die for and what I am passionate about. Basically, who God says I am. These define who I am, and it was not about where I am from, the color of my skin, my educational background, my family history and not even my past. When that light bulb popped, I finally knew who I was, and it was like everything finally made sense.

Knowing who you are is the best way to discover your true calling in life. Once you know who you are, you can choose or create work that is aligned with you. Your calling creates the work or opportunity that will make you feel both rewarded and fulfilled. That is exactly what happened in my life. After discovering who I am, the Lord revealed my purpose and my calling and yes, fear resurrected because I thought I wasn't worthy or good enough, I felt like I would have failed, I felt that I couldn't see the ending of my beginning but the word of God was my tower to eliminate fear and pursue what God told me to do.

Everyone wants to be the best version of themselves, but few do it. Many times, we are our own worst enemies and blockers when it comes to achieving success, chasing our dreams, and living a life that's filled with pursuit, passion and purpose. Many of us are filled with fear, doubt and self-destructive habits without realizing it, while others are aware, but lack the tools and/or knowledge in order to eliminate, modify and/or improve. After I knew what my assignment on Earth was, I knew I had to take steps to improve my public speaking, I needed advice from successful business owners to help me in my own businesses, I needed guidance to conduct my non-profit organization, I needed mentorship to help me carry out my passions and these made me to be who I am today.

Map to Mental Wellness

Here are a few tips to help you overcome your fears and fuel your success:

✦ Using Fear to Fuel Action

The most common reaction in a fearful situation is experiencing the feeling that you can't do it. Most times people get so accustomed to saying "I can't" without even attempting or trying. This fear of failure stops us from taking action and paralyzes us from moving forward. On the flip side, fear of failure can be a driving force towards success. For example, you fear failing an exam, so you would then make the necessary preparations to apply yourself properly to avoid failure. The preparations can come in the form of making a study schedule, take practice exams and if you are weak in certain areas, you seek the help you need. This way you use the fear to fuel your actions.

✦ Practice Makes Perfect

Confidence is who you are as a person and who you are comes from accepting who God says you are. Being confident reduces fear and over time, practicing confidence will make you perfect at what you do and what you are about. We have always heard this saying that, "Rome wasn't built in one day" and this is true. The good news is that once you face your fear by identifying what your fear is, the real cause of your fear, then you can combat the symptoms rather than shove it into a distant compartment of your brain, it begins losing the ability to rule you and dictate your decisions. Take the time to practice what combats your fear, and one day you will not be fearful anymore.

⚜ Confront Your Fears Immediately

Your ability to confront, deal with, and act despite your fears is the key to a happy, successful and purposeful life. One way you can practice confronting your fear is to identify a situation in your life of which you are afraid and resolve to deal with that fear situation immediately. Do not allow fear to control your happiness for another second. Resolve to confront the situation and put the fear behind you.

⚜ Move Toward the Fear

When you recognize a fear, you must discipline yourself to move towards it, as a result it grows smaller and more manageable. As your fears grow smaller, your confidence grows and your fears lose their control over you. Adversely, when you back away from a fear-inducing situation, your fear grows larger and larger. Shortly it dominates your thinking and feeling, preoccupies your entire being and takes control over your life.

In conclusion, fear is a very complicated emotion, but it can either motivate us or it can paralyze us depending on how we choose to approach it. As Christians, we must never allow it to dominate our lives, but use it to fuel our success and purpose.

Monique A. Lynch

Monique is a Programme Coordinator at the University of the West Indies, Mona Campus in Jamaica. She is also a woman of God, Youth Ambassador, Entrepreneur, Mental Health Advocate and the author of the books such as 'Betrayed', 'Building Your Confidence Workbook: A Guide for BBW', 'How to navigate a University: Perspectives of an undergraduate, graduate and staff/student' and 'An investigation into the increase of murder-suicide cases in Jamaica.'

As a professional, she has over 5 years of experience in the areas of business analysis, fund-raising and project management. Through her work, Monique has been able to manage and work on several projects that saw sustained development in the areas of education and mental health initiatives. Having recently completed her postgraduate studies in 2017 majoring in Mental Health, she decided to co-author this book to share her experience of how she used fear to fuel success and purpose in her life.

Contact Me: monique.a.lynch@gmail.com or chosenstarsfoundation@gmail.com.
Social media: IG: @chosenempress and FB:
@MoLynch4Change, @Chosenstarsfoundation

Chapter V.
Tarsha R. Lynch
911 What's your emergency?

**"Shall I bring to the time of birth, and not cause
delivery?" says the LORD.**
***"Shall I who causes delivery shut up the womb?"* says
your God. Isaiah 66:9 (NKJV)**

As I playback the mental video and epilogue in my head on
the countless times I heard that question 911 what's your
emergency? I can't help but to think of the grace, goodness,
and mercy of Jesus Christ. Unfortunately, I had been the
person on the other end of the phone in a crisis on multiple
occasions. Each time I could have lost my life. I could have
lost my life at the hands of assailants or I could have been a
victim of suicide or reverse homicide. It was in the late
2000's after a family violence assault, which I encountered
at the hands of my ex-husband that I first heard that chilling
question.

I could not believe that I survived the mean streets of Gary,
Indiana only to almost succumb to a domestic violence
assault. I was shocked, I was devasted and most of all I was
MAD. I was MAD as hell. I was bruised, broken mentality,
spiritually, emotionally, and financially. I was damaged
goods. I could not fathom for the life of me why my ex-
husband would want to slap me to the ground and try to

choke the life out of me. Yes, we had problems, what married couple didn't? He had reached his breaking point mentality. He was financially wounded due to child support garnishments that were making it hard for him to be the man he knew he was meant to be.

As for me, I was literally at the wrong place (at home) at the wrong time (bedtime). I watched him slip into almost a psychotic rage as I asked him questions about our finances and the issues with his previous marriage. One word led to another and before I knew it, I was on the floor fighting for my life. Shortly thereafter I was able to flee and call 911 for help. A few days later I began counseling and was diagnosed with PTSD. I couldn't believe the diagnosis. It was to my understanding that people only suffered from PTSD if they were in the war zone or near the front-line during war time.

I was given a series of medication to help me with my anxiety and to help me sleep. I was shame because of the diagnosis and the medication I had to take. I remember telling my cousin about the meds and she told me to take them for a while but not to become dependent on them. She told me to "pray" my way out of it. During this time in my life I wasn't suicidal, I was homicidal and angry that I couldn't repay him back for the damage he caused me. I looked at the bruises on my body and asked God how could YOU let this happen? Now I feel like I am having a heart attack every other day. As time progressed, I began to attend church and wing myself off of the anti-depressants. It took me about a year or more before I was able to resume my normal activity. I never thought to much about what happened as time went by. I had managed to suppress all emotions connected with the incident. About 2 years later, my now ex-husband and I went to counseling and put the pieces of our marriage back together. We stayed married for another 10 years and never had another physical altercation. We went to therapy a few times to try to hold onto the marriage but there was too much hurt and pain that could not be repaired. We remained cordial over the years and have since developed a 'sincere' bond.

The next time I would hear those words 911 what's your emergency would be in 2010. Me and my older sibling had gotten into a physical altercation about mismanagement of business funds. Once again, I was fighting for my life but this time I was in a position where I could have taken the life of my sibling. I had refused to be beaten again with the possibility of enforcing my fury. The blows I encountered to my head during this time could have killed me. I refused to die, I was MAD I had been assaulted before and barely escaped.

Round two of therapy and meds for PTSD. I told my doctor that I thought I was cured from PTSD. I really wasn't depressed and never (*admittedly*) suicidal so why did I have to be on this medicine and sit down to talk to someone? That seemed like a waste of money until one day it ALL hit me like a bag of rocks. I felt embarrassed and thought to myself why did God make me a punching bag? My favorite sibling had tried to beat me to a pulp. I felt like dying and giving up. Now I have scar in my scalp from the altercation to forever remind me of the trauma I endured for the rest of my natural life. I remember telling my mother how I felt, and she prayed for me and told me that it was going to be okay. She expressed how saddened and depressed she was about the incident. When my mother told me, she was depressed I felt even worse. She told me to keep my head up and keep going to therapy and taking the medicine. Again, I felt as though I didn't have the right to be depressed. Maybe I should have walked away instead of engaging in a heated argument that could have led to a loss of life or lives.

After a few months I picked myself up *again* in order to pursue life abundantly and to suppress my pain, my PTSD, and any ill feelings I was experiencing. I masked the pain with massive amounts of hard liquor and occasionally marijuana. I thought I was just being social. Everyone drinks and smokes a little bud every blue moon, right? This is the lie I told myself which allowed me to be okay with being an alcoholic. I had begun to drink so much that I almost wrecked my car on several occasions. Prompting those famous words 911 what's your emergency? This time I was in a ditch how I got there I have no idea. I was intoxicated and decided to drive home from an unknown area which caused me to use multiple freeways to get home. This was before the days of Uber and Lyft. I had no choice (so I thought) but to drive home.

Everyone I could have called to pick me up was out as well. Thanks to OnStar my location was determined and by the grace of GOD I was able to maneuver the car out of the ditch and arrive home safely without the police being dispatched. During that time, I didn't stop drinking and driving but I did stop drinking and driving long distances. I would reward myself cases of alcohol for making it through a hectic week and for being a 2x survivor of domestic violence. Whenever I would feel depressed, I would just fix me a couple of drinks or go out with my friends to get wasted. It felt completely normal. I didn't like going to therapy, taking pills and definitely didn't like being labeled PTSD. I stayed on this path of destruction for years. Masking my pain with alcohol and then sleeping pills. My alcoholic routine was so cold blooded I use to put Yaeger in my coffee a couple a times a week before going to work. Little did I know that years of suppressing my PTSD would cause more trauma.

Fast forward to the fall of 2017 when I made an abrupt decision to get into a relationship with a person who was a narcissist. This relationship took a tremendous toll on my soul as well as the life of my son Ben. The constant arguments, and verbal abuse almost pushed me over the edge. I felt helpless, and that it was my fault for excepting the relationship and allowing it to continue. It wasn't until it was halfway over that I learned the traits of a narcissist and the horrible trauma that suppressing my feelings over the years had caused. During this turbulent time, I kept hearing a small voice say, "trust the process". Every time I would hear this voice, I thought I was suffering from some form of psychosis. I would look at myself in the mirror and just scream. Every other week I wanted to die. I couldn't understand why God would allow me to lose my mind and to constantly be abused by the people I loved. It didn't seem fair. 911 what's your emergency? Rang in the atmosphere once again as I suffered from a panic attack that seemed to be a heart attack in the summer of 2018 due to stress of the turbulent relationship, I was in. The relationship had taken its final toll on me. What was this thing called life for? Who was God? Why was I still here? None of the things I endured made sense.

Map to Mental Wellness Success

I remember one-day while at work I decided to jump on YouTube and start listening to motivational speakers and church sermons. I wanted to live about 60/40 percent of the time. With the help of intercessory prayers and the shift of my mind I was able to come out from behind the mountain. It took less than a year for me to become the person I always knew myself to be at age 8. I did not think it was possible to pray, practice mediation, and make small lifestyle changes in-order to protect your mental health. Your mental health is your "Wealth".

We wash our bodies, brush our teeth, wash our clothes, wash our hair, and wash our cars. At what point is it imperative to wash your mind, your soul, and your spirituality? It seems so far-fetched until you "decide" that you want to live. I remember in the movie Menace to Society when Kane's grandfather asked him did, he want to live or die? Kane thought about it for a few minutes and replied I don't know. In August 2018 I asked myself that same question and unlike Kane I answered saying *YES*. If I desired to live, I must continue listening to the sermons and motivational speaking but how was I going to "live" if I only changed my mind but not my environment? A series of Godly orchestrated events caused my narcistic relationship to end. It was intense and abrupt as I didn't know if I was going to walk away alive.

I thought about 50 Cent's movie "Get Rich or Die Trying" in my head my new mantra became get to living or die trying and I did just that. I started by cutting alcohol of diet and began to fast for 12 hours per day 5-6 times per week while praying. As I stated earlier it began with a mindset shift and deciding to live. Not only did I decide to live, I decided to live life on my own terms. I decided that I was the author and the finisher of my life alongside God. I decided that no weapon formed against me could or would prosper. I decided I was the head and not the tail. I decided to accept the calling that God had put on my life once it was revealed to me. I used to look at people that lived harmoniously and abundantly and say wow they're blessed or wow they must have a lot of money. I used to say I wanted a life of abundance but after being a domestic violence survivor 2x it took any hope of that out of me for many years. I had accepted a life of mediocrity.

The face of depression and suicidal ideations or attempts is not a pretty one. There is no secret sauce to defeating depression. It all starts in the mind. People who suffer from mental illness must first decide to seek help and get tools for survival. It is a lifelong journey. I am here to tell you that you can make it. The thoughts and images in your mind are there to test your endurance. We all have gifts, but they are hard to discern when you aren't in a stable environment. They do work if they didn't there would not be millions of new coaches, and speakers on the scene screaming

"RENEW YOUR MIND". Win at the game of life by making mindset shifts. Tell yourself 100x times a day that you are more than conqueror, you were born to win and live a life of peace, prosperity, and fruitfulness.

When you are depressed do not suppress it or mask it. Consult with the national suicide hotline, church, friend or family if available. Start to think about the "life" you want to "live" and write down three things you could do to get to that life. Once you have successfully completed those 3 tasks, write down 3 more. Create a vision board and put it in a place where you can see it every day. Vision boards work (mine saved my life).

Give yourself a thousand second chances until you get it right. Most of all please do not give up. Let's make a pact to renew our minds daily by incorporating some form of spiritual or meditational cleansing into our routines and decide today to live.

Tarsha R. Lynch

Tarsha is a Gary, Indiana born native who relocated to Dallas, Texas in 1996. She is a mother of two adult children Amber and Benjamin and a grandmother to be. She is a multifaceted business professional and entrepreneur with several areas of certifications and licensing not limited to Texas Real Estate.

Tarsha has over 20 years of combined experience in the Real Estate and mortgage arenas. She is an active member of the Potter's House Dallas and a prior U.S. Military (Army Reservist), who holds an Associate of Business Management, Bachelor of Business Administration, and a Master's degree in Business Management. Tarsha is a mental health advocate, Godfidant Coach/Mentor & Forex Trader.

Find it out more about Tarsha @ www.iamtarshalynch.com and www.dashrealty.com.

Chapter IV.

Chante' Kiley-Washington

"Monster in the Dark"

Trust in The Lord with All Thine Heart and Lean Not to Your Own Understanding.
In All Thine Ways Acknowledge Him and He Shall Direct Thy Path…. Proverbs 3:5-6

ANOTHER DAY AND THE SAME CONVERSATION WITH MY MONSTER IN THE DARK…. GOD HELP ME PLEASE….

ME….
What in the world is wrong with me? Why do I not want to get out of bed? One minute I am eating everything around and the next minute I don't want to eat for days. What in the world is going on, I was fine yesterday! I was happy for no reason and it was just a good day without drugs and alcohol but today I feel like my world is in the pits! I do not feel like being bothered but I know I do not have a choice between the kids and work! Aw man, here I go…. Shower, clothes and the ever pleasant happy me. The people person that is always in a good mood and clowning in some form or fashion. The oldest child that was raised as a caregiver, nurturer and protector; all of me and my problems go on back burner. Raised in one of those households where much of nothing is discussed with the children i.e. mental health, sex

etc. etc. Oh yeah, let me not forget, **"WHAT GOES ON IN THIS HOUSE STAYS IN THIS HOUSE."** The one that must really have it all together, at least that is what it looks like on the outside to those that are not inside my circle, and I must live up to that expectation. I know what I can do, I can just make sure I stay busy from sunup to sundown, 24/7 and I will be alright.

MONSTER IN THE DARK:

Man, I will be glad when we get off, because all we need is
a pick me up.
It will make us feel better and give us energy.
We do not need to talk to anyone, we've been handling
things on
our own all this time, we're alright.
Talk to who? I wish we would talk to a shrink, so people
will say we are crazy.
Let alone they put us on some medicine and have us
walking around looking
like a zombie like those other people we see.
Please, nobody figured out anything is really wrong with us
yet,
so, we have been playing this off very well. It's just all in
our mind...
No-one will know we were drinking like crazy and getting
high.... We're good!
There is nothing wrong with putting a little bit of alcohol
and drugs in us to make us
feel a little bit better; Besides we have more fun like that
and everyone is doing it.

We are not hurting anyone. Don't worry about it, we are
just doing a little
bit more than we used to. We can handle it, we make
enough money,
we work hard, and besides, we need to take the edge off.
We are not like those people we see out there, homeless
and looking bad, we got this.

If any of this conversation sounds a little familiar, I am
going to suggest going to a professional and seek help
because the only wrong thing to do is to do nothing.

I was married twice and widowed twice. My first husband passed away from complications of cancer treatment. We were separated but we were still close and had a good friendship. It hurt me when he passed but I pulled myself together and put my strong face on and kept it moving. A few years later my high school sweetheart/ my daughter's father and I got back together. We had a thirty-five year on and off relationship. We were married on October 9, 2015 and he passed away from heart complications August 16, 2016; two months before our one-year anniversary. Every mask I had managed to use over the years just wasn't working for this tragedy. I lost it. I truly felt my sanity hanging on by a thread. It was so bad that my daughter had to put her grieving process on the back burner so she could deal with the family and his arrangements because I mentally and physically could not and she was my "Hero/Superwoman.". She kept me at her home for a long time because our (husband and me) apartment was not a good place for me to be.

Eventually, I returned to my apartment and that "Monster in the Dark" was not just making suggestions but had start barking orders at me. For instance. "Stay in bed we are not getting up as bad as we feel." I do not know how long in a weeks' time I went without bathing and/or eating. If the children would call to say they were coming over I would jump out of the bed, get cleaned up and find the appropriate mask to put on to convince them I was okay. Somedays that "Monster" tried to convince me it would be okay to join my husband because, my two children are grown and one of the two will take care of the younger one. That did not go over well with me so I opted to stay drunk every day. If it was not for God that would have spiraled into something ugly, which would had eventually resulted in death.

At some point I decided to just stay busy from the time I open my eyes to the time I could barely make it in the door. I later found out that is also a sign of Depression. I heard that from an author's story from another venue for Mental Health that was a part of Mrs. Venessa Anderson- Abrams' Ministry. I asked my Therapist if what I was doing also a sign of Depression.

"Please do not self-diagnose but if you believe something you have read sound similar/ familiar, PLEASE CONSULT A PROFESSIONAL THERAPIST/DOCTOR. Everyone does not have to experience such a tragedy as mine to make a mental health situation blow up. I found that I stayed in my Addiction so long due to denial. I also realized that self-medicating and denial of anything can lead to a very bad end result. I Thank God for the Prayers of friends, church family, family and most of all for God not letting me go.

Take everything serious when it comes to mental health, whether yours or someone else's.

My journey of pain from years of childhood traumas, "MY MONSTER IN THE DARK", which I just most recently as three years ago found out was Manic Depression and years of addiction lead me to my purpose of becoming an Addiction Counselor, Co-Author in this Anthology and an Advocate for Mental Health. What I was experiencing in my life is now known as Dual Diagnosis, but I did not know that then. Whatever you are experiencing, it is never too late to get help. Do not allow your circumstances define who you are or will be. I know that is easier said than done but nothing worth having is not worth fighting for. I had to fight myself with worrying about what people would think.

While I know God can do anything but fail, I also know He gave individuals gifts to help the next man. So, I went to God in prayer, then I went to a Therapist. It felt good to actually unloaded so much to someone else. I am so used to carrying everything and trying to save the world that I had lost me and was losing pieces of my sanity and did not want to acknowledge it. Yes, I take medication that helps with my Depression and it also helps me sleep. I come to learn that I cannot fulfill my purpose if I am not at my best.

Anyone that has survived some sort of trauma, dealt with mental health, substance abuse and/or a survivor of suicide/homicide/cancer whatever, either personally, close friend and/or family; It is your duty to stand up and fight....Fight to regain your life and help others fight for theirs....THAT IS YOUR PURPOSE AND MINE...BE BLESSED..

Map to Mental Health Wellness

My Map to Mental Health Wellness began with learning to go to God because I realized that nothing I was doing on my own worked. Second, I had to learn how to forgive myself. Forgive myself for all that I had done in my life, for all that I should have done and did not and forgive others for what they had done to me. Why? Because there is nothing, I could possibly do to change anything about my past. I had to learn that allowing myself to continue to stay in the midst of misery, dysfunction, anger, torment, codependent relationships, low self-esteem and not loving myself was only the Devils Playground where he was waiting for me to die in the midst of my misery and sins.

My next step was to learn to trust and talk to someone. I began talking to my closest and dearest friend/ sister which became a part of my support system. She is my accountability partner my sister girl, my vacation partner and my confidant. We know each other well enough to say, "Hey, what is going on with you?" Building a strong support system is the next most valuable thing next to having God in my life. Why? Because as long as things are held inside and allowed to grow, it will blow up and more times than not, it will not be in a good way. Find someone to trust, that will not be judgmental and who have your best interest at heart and let it all spill out. If there is no one in your personal life, get a Therapist. I am fortunate enough to have both. Guess what, if there is no one God is always on the Throne and he will not tell anyone or be judgmental.

My third step which actually came in with the other steps as well and that is to come out of "Denial." I am not that super strong, nothing ever wrong, the world is always roses, there is nothing wrong with me. Yes, I had to come to grips with the fact I have a Mental Health Diagnosis. I had to want to deal with that in a functional manner and that is to take my medication and visit with my Therapist. Am I perfect at keeping my appointments? Absolutely not! But I now know that if I do not want to go back where I was, I have to stay on top of it. Do not worry about what others may think. Actually, no one will know unless you tell it. Mmmm, food for thought. I also had to learn that I am "Human" and I need to learn my limitations with some things but I also keep forefront; "I Can Do All Things Through Christ Who Strengthens Me."
Philippians 4:13

Last but not least. Surround yourself with "Positive People." Network, attend various workshops, there is no telling what may happen once you attend. Look at me for example. I always wanted to be a writer and to tell my story. On a humble, I attended a workshop that was held by Ms. Venessa and the rest is History. Look at God at Work......

"CHANGE WILL NEVER COME IF CHANGE IS NOT PUT IN PLACE!!!"
Mrs. Chante' Kiley- Washington

Chante' Kiley- Washington

Chante' is the mother of three adult children and three grandchildren. Chante' received her Associates of Science Degree from Baltimore City Community College. She then pursued and received her Bachelors of Science Degree from Coppin State University; where she began the Master's Program.

Chante' chose to pursue her career as an Addiction Counselor due to her own personal life experiences. She is currently an Addiction Counselor at New Vision House of Hope located in Downtown Baltimore. Chante' loves her career because it is her mission to share knowledge, thus creating power in others. She has learned a very important fact about herself; the fact that a Mental Health Diagnosis was the Monster in the Dark that contributed to her self-medication in her past life. With help from God and Professionals, Chante' can choose to do better because she now knows better. She also realizes that it is never too late to get help.

Email Chante: Chantekiley1@gmail.com

If you interested in sharing your story and being *"A VOICE"* for those that are afraid to speak due to the shame, stigma and suffering associated with mental illness, please contact us TODAY at:
www.sd-ppp.org **OR** stopsuicide@sd-ppp.com.

May you be WELL Holistically.

Peace and Blessings,

Venessa

Mental Health Resources
Dial 911 when in immediate danger!

American Foundation for Suicide Prevention
www.afsp.org

American Psychological Association
www.apa.org

Behavior Healthlink
www.behavioralhealthlink.com

Center for Disease Control
www.cdc.gov

National Alliance on Mental Illness
www.nami.org

Mental Health America
www.mentalhealthamerica.net

Self-Discovery: Pain, Positioning & Purpose, Inc.
www.sd-ppp.org

Suicide Prevention Lifeline
www.suicidepreventionlifeline.org

Substance Abuse and Mental Health Services
Administration
www.samhsa.gov

The Respect Institute

www.dbhdd.georgia.gov

Viewpoint Health

https://www.myviewpointhealth.org/

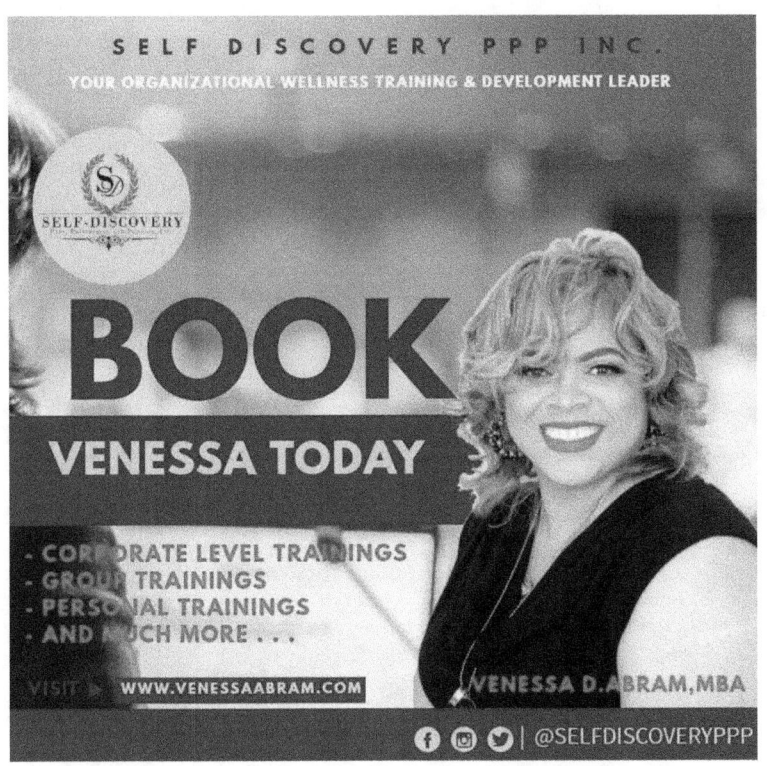

For Bookings, please visit
www.sd-ppp.org

Self-Discovery is a Daily
Journey!